NATURAL REMEDIES TO ALL DISEASE

Comprehensive Guide to Natural Cure For All Disease Using Nature's Resources and Herbal Remedies For Healing Without Pills

Dr. Fredrick Kim

TABLE OF CONTENTS

INTRODUCTION TO NATURAL REMEDIES

Natural remedies have been used for centuries across cultures as a way to support health, treat common ailments, and promote overall wellness. Rooted in the use of plants, minerals, and lifestyle practices, these remedies focus on utilizing nature's resources to aid in healing and prevention without synthetic drugs. With a growing interest in holistic health and alternative medicine, natural remedies continue to gain popularity as safe, accessible, and often effective solutions to many health issues.

What are Natural Remedies?

Natural remedies refer to treatments derived from natural sources—mainly plants (herbs), minerals, and organic substances—that are used to alleviate symptoms or improve health. Unlike pharmaceuticals, which are often synthetic, natural remedies come in their purest forms and are minimally processed. Examples include herbal teas, essential oils, vitamins, minerals, and foods rich in medicinal properties. Natural remedies can be used for common ailments like colds and digestive issues, as well as chronic conditions such as high blood pressure and joint pain.

Benefits of Natural Remedies

Fewer Side Effects: Since natural remedies are derived from whole foods and plants, they generally have fewer side effects than synthetic drugs, making them safer for long-term use.

Holistic Approach: Natural remedies focus on treating the whole body, not just symptoms, often addressing root causes like inflammation, immunity, or stress.

Cost-Effective: Many natural remedies, such as ginger, garlic, and aloe vera, are inexpensive and readily available.

Environmentally Friendly: Using natural, locally-sourced remedies reduces the environmental impact of manufacturing synthetic drugs.

Empowerment in Self-Care: Natural remedies can provide a sense of self-sufficiency, as people can take a more active role in their health and wellness.

Precautions and Safety Tips
While natural remedies are generally safe, it's essential to use them wisely:

Consult Healthcare Providers: Some natural remedies may interact with medications or may not be suitable for certain conditions.

Use Proper Dosage: Even natural remedies can have side effects or cause harm if used in excess.

Choose Quality Sources: Organic and reputable sources are best for ensuring the purity and potency of remedies.

Understand Limitations: Natural remedies can be helpful for mild to moderate issues, but serious conditions may require conventional medical treatments.

The Philosophy Behind Natural Remedies
Natural medicine is often rooted in traditions such as Ayurveda, Traditional Chinese Medicine, and
Native American healing practices. These systems emphasize balance, prevention, and lifestyle as fundamental aspects of health. By focusing on balance—whether through diet, exercise, mental well-being, or herbal support—natural

remedies aim to help the body restore its natural equilibrium. This philosophy views health as a state of physical, emotional, and spiritual harmony rather than merely the absence of disease.

How to Get Started with Natural Remedies
Identify Your Needs: Start by assessing any specific health concerns or goals, such as boosting immunity, improving digestion, or reducing anxiety.

Research Remedies: Look into trusted sources, consult guides, and consider seeking advice from a qualified naturopath or herbalist.

Incorporate Gradually: Begin with a few simple remedies, like herbal teas or essential oils, and monitor your body's response.

Focus on Lifestyle: Natural remedies work best when paired with healthy habits, including a balanced diet, regular exercise, and stress management.

Natural remedies are not a cure-all, but they offer a gentle, supportive way to improve health and prevent illness. When used responsibly, they can complement conventional treatments and help nurture a well-rounded approach to health.

CHAPTER 1
Immune System Boosters

A strong immune system is essential for fighting off infections, protecting the body from harmful invaders, and maintaining overall health. There are several natural remedies and lifestyle practices that can enhance immune function, reduce the duration of illnesses, and improve resilience against pathogens. Here are some of the most effective immune system boosters:

Elderberry (Sambucus nigra)
Benefits: Elderberry has powerful antiviral and antioxidant properties that support immune health. It's particularly effective against cold and flu viruses and is thought to reduce the severity and duration of symptoms.

How to Use: Elderberry can be consumed as a syrup, supplement, or tea. Be cautious about the dosage and use only reputable products, as raw elderberries can be toxic.

Echinacea
Benefits: Echinacea is an herb known for stimulating immune activity. Studies suggest it may increase white blood cell count, which helps the body fight infections.

How to Use: Echinacea can be taken in capsule form, as a tea, or as a tincture. It's best used at the onset of cold or flu symptoms to reduce duration and severity.

Vitamin C
Benefits: Vitamin C is a well-known immune booster with antioxidant properties. It supports white blood cell function, enhances the body's ability to produce antibodies, and protects cells from oxidative stress.

Sources: Citrus fruits (oranges, lemons, grapefruits), bell peppers, strawberries, and broccoli are rich in vitamin C. Supplements are also available.

How to Use: For immune support, aim to get vitamin C through food sources daily or take a supplement of 500-1,000 mg if needed.

Probiotics

Benefits: Probiotics are beneficial bacteria that support gut health, which is closely linked to immune function. A healthy gut microbiome strengthens the immune system by preventing the growth of harmful bacteria and promoting balanced immune responses.

Sources: Yogurt, kefir, sauerkraut, kimchi, and kombucha are good sources of probiotics.

How to Use: Consume probiotic-rich foods daily, or consider taking a probiotic supplement to maintain gut health and boost immunity.

Garlic

Benefits: Garlic contains a compound called allicin, which has antimicrobial, antiviral, and immune-boosting effects. Regular consumption of garlic can help lower the risk of getting sick.

How to Use: Use raw or lightly cooked garlic in meals or take a garlic supplement. Crushing or chopping garlic activates its beneficial compounds.

Zinc

Benefits: Zinc is an essential mineral that plays a critical role in immune cell function and helps reduce the duration of colds. It also acts as an antioxidant, protecting cells from damage.

Sources: Foods rich in zinc include pumpkin seeds, lentils, chickpeas, beans, and nuts. Supplements are also available, particularly useful during cold and flu season.

How to Use: A daily intake of 8-11 mg for adults is generally recommended, but supplements up to 25 mg can be taken during illness.

Ginger

Benefits: Ginger has potent anti-inflammatory and antioxidant effects that support immune health and may help relieve symptoms of colds, such as sore throat and congestion.

How to Use: Fresh ginger can be added to tea, smoothies, or meals. Ginger tea with honey and lemon is especially beneficial for immune support and soothing sore throats.

Turmeric (Curcumin)

Benefits: Curcumin, the active compound in turmeric, is a strong antioxidant with anti-inflammatory effects. It helps modulate immune responses and protect against chronic inflammation, which can weaken immunity.

How to Use: Add turmeric to food, make turmeric tea, or take a curcumin supplement. Combining turmeric with black pepper enhances absorption.

Green Tea

Benefits: Green tea contains catechins, powerful antioxidants that support the immune system. It also contains L-theanine, an amino acid that may help immune cells fight off pathogens.

How to Use: Drink 1-3 cups of green tea daily for immune support and added antioxidant benefits.

Mushrooms (Reishi, Shiitake, Maitake)
Benefits: Medicinal mushrooms, such as reishi, shiitake, and maitake, contain beta-glucans that enhance immune response by activating immune cells. Reishi, in particular, is also known to reduce stress, which can benefit immunity.

How to Use: Incorporate these mushrooms into soups or stir-fries, or take them as supplements in capsule or powder form.

Sleep and Stress Management
Benefits: Quality sleep and effective stress management are vital for optimal immune function. Lack of sleep and chronic stress suppress immune responses, making the body more susceptible to illness.

How to Use: Aim for 7-8 hours of sleep each night and practice stress-reduction techniques, such as mindfulness meditation, yoga, or deep breathing exercises.

Hydration
Benefits: Staying well-hydrated supports immune health by helping to flush out toxins and ensuring cells function properly.

How to Use: Drink at least 8 glasses of water daily, and consider herbal teas for added immune support. Herbal teas, like ginger, peppermint, or chamomile, also provide hydration and additional immune benefits.

Tips for Optimal Immune Support
Balanced Diet: A diet rich in fruits, vegetables, lean proteins, and whole grains provides essential nutrients to support immunity.

Exercise Regularly: Moderate exercise can boost immune function and reduce inflammation.
Avoid Smoking and Excessive Alcohol: Both can weaken the immune system and increase susceptibility to infections.

Incorporating these immune-boosting remedies and lifestyle habits into your routine can strengthen your immune system and help keep illnesses at bay. Natural immune support is most effective when combined with a balanced diet, good hygiene, and regular health check-ups.

CHAPTER 2
Cold and Flu Relief

Colds and flu are common, especially during colder months, and while they are typically mild, their symptoms can be uncomfortable. Natural remedies can ease symptoms, speed up recovery, and strengthen immunity to prevent future infections. Here are some effective ways to find relief from cold and flu symptoms:

Ginger Tea
Benefits: Ginger has powerful anti-inflammatory and antiviral properties, making it effective for soothing sore throats, reducing congestion, and fighting viruses.
How to Use: Slice fresh ginger and steep in hot water for 10 minutes. Add honey and lemon for added benefits. Drink up to three times a day.

Honey and Lemon
Benefits: Honey coats the throat, reducing irritation and coughing, while lemon provides vitamin C and antioxidants to boost immunity.
How to Use: Mix one tablespoon of honey with the juice of half a lemon in warm water. Sip this mixture throughout the day for throat relief and hydration.

Garlic
Benefits: Garlic contains allicin, a compound with strong antimicrobial properties that help fight colds and flu viruses. It's also a natural immune booster.
How to Use: Crush or chop raw garlic and let it sit for a few minutes to activate allicin. Add it to food, or mix crushed garlic with honey and consume a small spoonful.

Elderberry

Benefits: Elderberry has antiviral and immune-boosting properties, making it a popular choice for shortening the duration of cold and flu symptoms.
How to Use: Elderberry syrup or supplements can be taken at the onset of symptoms. Dosage varies by product, so follow package instructions.

Echinacea

Benefits: Echinacea is known for stimulating the immune system and can help reduce the severity and length of cold symptoms if taken early.
How to Use: Take echinacea as a tea, tincture, or capsule at the first sign of illness. Use it for short periods to avoid tolerance.

Steam Inhalation

Benefits: Inhaling steam helps to relieve nasal congestion and soothe irritated respiratory passages.
How to Use: Boil water and pour it into a bowl. Lean over the bowl with a towel over your head to trap the steam, and inhale deeply for 5-10 minutes. Adding eucalyptus oil enhances the decongesting effect.

Warm Saltwater Gargle

Benefits: Saltwater helps reduce throat inflammation, kill bacteria, and ease throat soreness.
How to Use: Dissolve half a teaspoon of salt in warm water and gargle for 30 seconds. Repeat several times a day as needed.

Peppermint Tea

Benefits: Peppermint contains menthol, which helps to thin mucus and relieve nasal congestion. Its antimicrobial and antioxidant properties also aid in cold relief.

How to Use: Steep peppermint tea bags or fresh peppermint leaves in hot water. Drink a few cups daily to clear sinuses and reduce headaches.

Turmeric and Honey Paste

Benefits: Turmeric's active compound, curcumin, has anti-inflammatory and antiviral properties, and honey coats and soothes the throat.

How to Use: Mix half a teaspoon of turmeric powder with a teaspoon of honey. Take this mixture once or twice a day to ease coughing and boost immunity.

Probiotics

Benefits: Probiotics promote healthy gut bacteria, which play a crucial role in immune health. A healthy gut microbiome can help the body fight off infections more effectively.

Sources: Yogurt, kefir, and other fermented foods like sauerkraut and kimchi are good sources of probiotics. You can also take a probiotic supplement.

Rest and Hydration

Benefits: Adequate rest allows your body to focus on fighting off the infection. Hydration helps thin mucus, soothe sore throats, and prevent dehydration.

How to Use: Aim for at least 7-8 hours of sleep, and drink plenty of fluids, including water, herbal teas, and clear broths. Avoid caffeine and alcohol, as they can dehydrate the body.

Zinc Supplements

Benefits: Zinc is essential for immune function and can help reduce the severity and duration of cold symptoms if taken at the onset of symptoms.

How to Use: Zinc lozenges or supplements are effective when taken within 24 hours of the first symptoms. Follow recommended dosage on the product label.

Chicken Soup

Benefits: A classic remedy, chicken soup provides warmth, hydration, and nutrients. The broth's anti-inflammatory effect may help reduce upper respiratory symptoms.

How to Use: Prepare or buy a low-sodium chicken soup, ideally with vegetables like garlic, onions, and carrots for added nutrients. Enjoy warm throughout the day for comfort and hydration.

Apple Cider Vinegar

Benefits: Apple cider vinegar helps alkalize the body and contains probiotics to support immune health. It can also thin mucus and relieve sinus congestion.

How to Use: Mix one tablespoon of apple cider vinegar in warm water and drink once or twice daily. Add honey for added soothing effects.

Essential Oils for Diffusion

Benefits: Essential oils like eucalyptus, peppermint, and tea tree oil have antimicrobial properties and help relieve congestion.

How to Use: Add a few drops of essential oil to a diffuser, or mix with a carrier oil and rub it on your chest to clear sinuses and ease breathing.

Tips for Preventing Cold and Flu

Practice Good Hygiene: Wash hands frequently and avoid touching your face.

Eat Immune-Boosting Foods: A balanced diet rich in vitamins and antioxidants strengthens your immune defenses.

Stay Warm and Avoid Stress: Cold weather can suppress the immune system, so dressing warmly and managing stress is essential for prevention.

Natural remedies are most effective when used early in the course of a cold or flu and can be safely combined with other practices, like getting enough rest and staying hydrated. For persistent or severe symptoms, consult a healthcare provider.

CHAPTER 3
High Blood Pressure Management

High blood pressure (hypertension) is a common condition that can lead to serious health problems like heart disease and stroke if left unmanaged. Many natural remedies and lifestyle adjustments can help reduce blood pressure levels, often complementing prescribed treatments. Here are effective natural methods for managing high blood pressure:

Garlic
Benefits: Garlic has been shown to have blood-pressure-lowering effects due to a compound called allicin, which helps relax blood vessels.
How to Use: Eat 1-2 cloves of raw garlic daily, add it to meals, or take a garlic supplement. Crushing garlic activates its beneficial compounds.

Hibiscus Tea
Benefits: Hibiscus tea is rich in antioxidants and acts as a natural diuretic, helping reduce blood pressure by relaxing blood vessels and increasing urine output.
How to Use: Steep dried hibiscus flowers in hot water for 5-10 minutes and drink 1-2 cups daily. Avoid if pregnant, as it may stimulate uterine contractions.

Omega-3 Fatty Acids
Benefits: Omega-3s have anti-inflammatory and vasodilating effects, which help lower blood pressure. They also support overall cardiovascular health.
Sources: Fatty fish (salmon, mackerel, sardines), flaxseeds, chia seeds, and walnuts. Fish oil supplements are also available.
How to Use: Aim to consume fatty fish 2-3 times a week or take a fish oil supplement as directed.

Dark Chocolate (70% Cocoa or Higher)

Benefits: Dark chocolate contains flavonoids, which help dilate blood vessels and improve blood flow, thereby lowering blood pressure.

How to Use: Eat a small piece (1 oz.) of dark chocolate daily to help support heart health.

Potassium-Rich Foods

Benefits: Potassium helps balance sodium levels in the body, reducing strain on blood vessels and helping lower blood pressure.

Sources: Bananas, oranges, sweet potatoes, tomatoes, avocados, and leafy greens.

How to Use: Include potassium-rich foods in your daily diet to help manage blood pressure naturally.

Magnesium

Benefits: Magnesium helps regulate blood pressure by relaxing blood vessels. A deficiency in magnesium may lead to higher blood pressure.

Sources: Leafy green vegetables, nuts (especially almonds and cashews), seeds, whole grains, and beans.

How to Use: Ensure a balanced intake of magnesium through diet, or consider a supplement if needed, with the guidance of a healthcare provider.

Apple Cider Vinegar (ACV)

Benefits: Apple cider vinegar is thought to help lower blood pressure by improving blood circulation and promoting detoxification.

How to Use: Mix one tablespoon of ACV with a glass of water and drink daily. Be sure to rinse your mouth afterward, as ACV is acidic and can erode tooth enamel.

Beetroot Juice

Benefits: Beetroot is high in nitrates, which help dilate blood vessels and improve blood flow, lowering blood pressure.

How to Use: Drink a glass of fresh beetroot juice daily. If the taste is too strong, mix it with carrot or apple juice for sweetness.

Coenzyme Q10 (CoQ10)

Benefits: CoQ10 is an antioxidant that supports cardiovascular health and can help lower blood pressure by improving blood vessel function.

How to Use: CoQ10 supplements are available in most health stores. The typical dosage ranges from 100-200 mg per day.

Celery Seed

Benefits: Celery seed extract has a diuretic effect and contains compounds that help relax blood vessels, which can reduce blood pressure.

How to Use: Celery seed supplements are available, or you can include celery in your diet. Consult a healthcare provider before using celery seed supplements if you are on other blood pressure medications.

Pomegranate Juice

Benefits: Pomegranate juice is high in antioxidants and has been shown to lower blood pressure, particularly systolic blood pressure.

How to Use: Drink a small glass (4-8 oz.) of unsweetened pomegranate juice daily. Check with your healthcare provider if you're on blood pressure medications, as pomegranate juice can interact with certain drugs.

Meditation and Deep Breathing

Benefits: Meditation and deep breathing exercises help activate the body's relaxation response, reducing stress hormones and blood pressure.

How to Use: Practice deep breathing exercises or meditation for 5-10 minutes daily. Apps or guided videos can be helpful.

Regular Exercise
Benefits: Physical activity strengthens the heart, helps control weight, and reduces stress, all of which contribute to lower blood pressure.
How to Use: Aim for at least 30 minutes of moderate exercise (such as walking, cycling, or swimming) most days of the week.

Reduce Salt Intake
Benefits: Excess sodium can increase blood pressure by causing the body to retain water, adding pressure to blood vessels.
How to Use: Limit processed and packaged foods, which are often high in sodium, and use herbs or spices instead of salt to season food. Aim for no more than 1,500-2,300 mg of sodium per day.

Limit Alcohol and Caffeine
Benefits: Both alcohol and caffeine can raise blood pressure temporarily and, in excess, can lead to long-term hypertension.
How to Use: Limit alcohol to one drink per day for women and two for men, and reduce caffeine intake, especially if you're sensitive to its effects on blood pressure.

Manage Stress
Benefits: Chronic stress can increase blood pressure by causing the body to produce stress hormones like cortisol and adrenaline.

How to Use: Practice stress management techniques such as yoga, tai chi, or engaging in hobbies. Regular relaxation can help lower blood pressure over time.

Tips for Success with Natural Blood Pressure Management

Track Your Blood Pressure: Regular monitoring can help you see the effects of lifestyle changes and adjust as needed.

Adopt a Balanced Diet: A diet like the DASH (Dietary Approaches to Stop Hypertension) diet emphasizes fruits, vegetables, whole grains, lean protein, and low-fat dairy to naturally support blood pressure.

Stay Hydrated: Proper hydration helps balance electrolytes and supports healthy blood vessel function.

Using these natural remedies and lifestyle strategies can be an effective way to manage high blood pressure. For best results, combine these approaches with regular check-ups and follow your healthcare provider's recommendations.

CHAPTER 4
Digestive Health

Maintaining a healthy digestive system is crucial for overall well-being, as it impacts nutrient absorption, energy levels, immunity, and even mood. Many natural remedies and lifestyle habits can improve digestion, reduce symptoms like bloating and constipation, and promote a balanced gut microbiome. Here are effective ways to support digestive health:

Probiotics
Benefits: Probiotics are beneficial bacteria that help balance gut flora, improving digestion and reducing issues like bloating, gas, and constipation.
Sources: Yogurt, kefir, sauerkraut, kimchi, miso, and kombucha.
How to Use: Include a serving of probiotic-rich foods daily, or consider a probiotic supplement for added support.

Fiber-Rich Foods
Benefits: Dietary fiber promotes regular bowel movements, prevents constipation, and feeds beneficial gut bacteria. Soluble fiber (found in oats, apples, and beans) absorbs water to soften stool, while insoluble fiber (found in whole grains and vegetables) adds bulk to stool.
Sources: Fruits, vegetables, whole grains, legumes, nuts, and seeds.
How to Use: Aim for 25-30 grams of fiber daily, gradually increasing your intake to avoid bloating.

Ginger
Benefits: Ginger stimulates digestive enzymes, aids in stomach emptying, and can alleviate nausea, bloating, and indigestion.

How to Use: Add fresh ginger to meals, make ginger tea, or take a ginger supplement before meals to support digestion.

Peppermint

Benefits: Peppermint has antispasmodic properties that relax the muscles of the gastrointestinal tract, making it effective for reducing gas, bloating, and symptoms of irritable bowel syndrome (IBS).

How to Use: Drink peppermint tea after meals or take enteric-coated peppermint oil capsules to prevent acid reflux.

Apple Cider Vinegar (ACV)

Benefits: ACV may improve digestion by increasing stomach acidity, which helps break down food more efficiently and prevents indigestion and bloating.

How to Use: Mix one tablespoon of ACV in a glass of water and drink before meals. Be sure to rinse your mouth afterward to protect tooth enamel.

Stay Hydrated

Benefits: Water helps soften stool and prevents constipation. Proper hydration is essential for smooth digestion and nutrient absorption.

How to Use: Aim for 8 glasses of water a day. Herbal teas and water-rich fruits and vegetables like cucumber and watermelon also help with hydration.

Fennel Seeds

Benefits: Fennel seeds contain compounds that relax the digestive tract and reduce gas and bloating.

How to Use: Chew on a small amount of fennel seeds after meals or make fennel tea by steeping the seeds in hot water.

Turmeric

Benefits: Curcumin, the active compound in turmeric, has anti-inflammatory properties that may benefit digestive health and relieve symptoms of digestive disorders.
How to Use: Add turmeric to food or make a turmeric tea. Pair with black pepper to enhance absorption of curcumin.

Digestive Enzymes

Benefits: Digestive enzymes help break down food into nutrients, which improves digestion and reduces bloating and gas.
How to Use: You can find digestive enzyme supplements, or consume foods like pineapple (rich in bromelain) and papaya (rich in papain) that naturally contain enzymes.

Aloe Vera Juice

Benefits: Aloe vera has anti-inflammatory properties and may help relieve symptoms of acid reflux, soothe the digestive tract, and support regular bowel movements.
How to Use: Drink a small amount of aloe vera juice (1-2 oz.) diluted in water. Start with a small dose to ensure it doesn't cause diarrhea.

Chamomile Tea

Benefits: Chamomile has anti-inflammatory and muscle-relaxing effects that can ease digestive discomfort, reduce gas, and soothe an upset stomach.
How to Use: Steep chamomile tea for 5-10 minutes and drink it after meals to promote digestion and relaxation.

Regular Exercise

Benefits: Physical activity stimulates the muscles of the digestive tract, promoting regular bowel movements and reducing bloating.
How to Use: Aim for at least 30 minutes of exercise daily. Walking after meals can also aid digestion.

Limit Processed Foods and Sugar

Benefits: Processed foods and sugar can disrupt the gut microbiome, leading to digestive issues like bloating, gas, and constipation.

How to Use: Focus on whole foods like fruits, vegetables, lean proteins, and whole grains, and limit sugary and highly processed foods.

Avoid Overeating and Eat Mindfully

Benefits: Eating too much at once can overwhelm the digestive system, leading to indigestion and bloating. Mindful eating helps improve digestion by promoting slower, more thorough chewing.

How to Use: Eat smaller, more frequent meals and take time to chew thoroughly. Avoid distractions like phones or TV while eating.

Prebiotic Foods

Benefits: Prebiotics are types of fiber that feed beneficial gut bacteria, helping them thrive and support digestion.

Sources: Bananas, onions, garlic, leeks, asparagus, and oats.

How to Use: Include prebiotic-rich foods in your diet regularly to support a healthy gut microbiome.

Avoid Drinking Too Much Water with Meals

Benefits: Drinking excessive water with meals may dilute stomach acid, which is essential for breaking down food.

How to Use: Try to drink most of your water between meals rather than during meals to allow your digestive enzymes to function optimally.

Manage Stress

Benefits: Chronic stress can negatively affect digestion, leading to issues like IBS and indigestion.

How to Use: Practice relaxation techniques like meditation, deep breathing exercises, or yoga to reduce stress and improve digestion.

Try Intermittent Fasting
Benefits: Intermittent fasting can give the digestive system a break, reduce inflammation, and promote gut health by allowing beneficial bacteria to flourish.
How to Use: Consider a fasting method, like the 16/8 method (fasting for 16 hours, eating within an 8-hour window). Consult with a healthcare provider if you have any digestive issues.

Tips for a Healthy Digestive System
Chew Thoroughly: Digestion begins in the mouth, so chewing food thoroughly aids the digestive process.

Avoid Late-Night Eating: Eating late at night can lead to acid reflux and disrupt digestive function.
Get Enough Sleep: Poor sleep can worsen digestive health, so aim for 7-8 hours of quality sleep each night.

Adopting these natural remedies and lifestyle adjustments can significantly improve your digestive health and help prevent digestive issues. For persistent or severe symptoms, consult a healthcare provider.

CHAPTER 5
Joint Pain and Arthritis Relief

Joint pain and arthritis affect many people, impacting quality of life and mobility. While medications can provide relief, natural remedies and lifestyle changes can also help manage symptoms, reduce inflammation, and improve joint function. Here are some effective ways to relieve joint pain and manage arthritis naturally:

Turmeric and Curcumin

Benefits: Curcumin, the active compound in turmeric, has strong anti-inflammatory properties that can help reduce joint pain and stiffness.

How to Use: Take a turmeric supplement with black pepper (for better absorption) or add turmeric to your daily meals. Aim for 500-1,000 mg of curcumin per day.

Ginger

Benefits: Ginger has anti-inflammatory effects that may help relieve arthritis pain by reducing inflammatory markers in the body.

How to Use: Add fresh ginger to meals, make ginger tea, or take ginger supplements as directed. It can also be used topically in the form of a ginger-infused oil for direct application on sore joints.

Omega-3 Fatty Acids

Benefits: Omega-3s reduce inflammation and may help reduce joint pain and stiffness, particularly for people with rheumatoid arthritis.

Sources: Fatty fish like salmon, mackerel, and sardines, as well as flaxseeds, chia seeds, and walnuts.

How to Use: Aim for 2-3 servings of fatty fish per week or consider taking a high-quality fish oil supplement.

Epsom Salt Baths

Benefits: Epsom salt contains magnesium, which helps relax muscles and reduce joint pain.

How to Use: Add 1-2 cups of Epsom salt to a warm bath and soak for 15-20 minutes. Repeat a few times a week for relief.

Capsaicin Cream

Benefits: Capsaicin, derived from chili peppers, temporarily reduces pain by blocking pain signals in the body.

How to Use: Apply a capsaicin cream to the affected joints a few times a day. Be cautious, as it can cause a burning sensation. Avoid contact with eyes and wash hands after applying.

Boswellia Serrata (Indian Frankincense)

Benefits: Boswellia has anti-inflammatory effects that can improve joint health and reduce pain and stiffness, particularly in osteoarthritis.

How to Use: Boswellia supplements are available in capsule form. A common dose is 300-400 mg, taken two to three times daily.

Glucosamine and Chondroitin

Benefits: Glucosamine and chondroitin are natural compounds found in cartilage that may help slow cartilage breakdown and improve joint function.

How to Use: Take 1,500 mg of glucosamine and 1,200 mg of chondroitin daily, as directed. It may take several weeks to feel the full effects.

Heat and Cold Therapy

Benefits: Applying heat relaxes muscles and eases stiffness, while cold reduces inflammation and numbs sharp pain.

How to Use: Use a heating pad for 15-20 minutes or a cold pack for 10-15 minutes on the affected area. Alternate as needed to reduce symptoms.

Vitamin D and Calcium

Benefits: Vitamin D helps with calcium absorption and plays a crucial role in maintaining bone health, which is essential for supporting joints.

Sources: Sun exposure, fortified dairy products, leafy greens, and supplements.

How to Use: Get 15-20 minutes of sunlight daily or consider a supplement. Many people with arthritis are deficient in vitamin D.

Green Tea

Benefits: Green tea contains antioxidants, including EGCG, which reduce inflammation and can slow the destruction of cartilage in joints.

How to Use: Drink 1-2 cups of green tea daily, or consider green tea extract if you prefer supplements.

Exercise and Physical Therapy

Benefits: Regular, low-impact exercise strengthens muscles around joints, reduces stiffness, and improves flexibility.

Types of Exercise: Walking, swimming, cycling, and gentle yoga. Physical therapy can provide tailored exercises to build strength and improve joint function.

How to Use: Aim for at least 30 minutes of low-impact exercise most days of the week. Consult a physical therapist for customized exercises if needed.

Anti-Inflammatory Diet

Benefits: An anti-inflammatory diet, rich in whole foods, fruits, vegetables, and healthy fats, can help reduce overall inflammation and joint pain.

Key Foods: Leafy greens, berries, nuts, seeds, olive oil, and fatty fish. Avoid processed foods, sugary drinks, and red meat, which can increase inflammation.

Massage Therapy
Benefits: Massage can improve circulation, reduce stiffness, and relieve pain by relaxing the muscles around the joints.
How to Use: Seek a trained massage therapist who has experience with arthritis, or use a gentle massage oil to self-massage sore areas.

Willow Bark
Benefits: Willow bark has natural anti-inflammatory and pain-relieving properties, similar to aspirin.
How to Use: Willow bark is available as a tea, powder, or supplement. Follow dosing instructions, and consult with a healthcare provider if you're on other medications.

Acupuncture
Benefits: Acupuncture can help reduce pain and inflammation by stimulating specific points in the body, improving blood flow, and releasing endorphins.
How to Use: Seek a licensed acupuncturist and discuss your symptoms and areas of pain. Several sessions may be needed for full benefits.

Bone Broth
Benefits: Bone broth contains glucosamine, chondroitin, collagen, and amino acids that support joint health and reduce inflammation.
How to Use: Drink 1-2 cups of bone broth daily or use it in cooking. It's also available in powder form for easy use.

Tips for Managing Joint Pain and Arthritis
Maintain a Healthy Weight: Excess weight puts additional stress on joints, particularly in the knees, hips, and spine.

Stay Hydrated: Water keeps joints lubricated, reducing friction and pain.
Get Enough Rest: Quality sleep helps repair tissues and reduces inflammation.
Avoid High-Impact Activities: Stick to low-impact exercises to avoid joint strain.
Using these natural remedies and lifestyle changes can significantly improve joint health and help manage arthritis symptoms.

CHAPTER 6
Anxiety and Sleep Disorders

Anxiety and sleep disorders are often interconnected, as one can exacerbate the other. Managing anxiety can improve sleep quality, while better sleep can help reduce anxiety. Here are natural remedies and lifestyle tips to manage anxiety, promote relaxation, and improve sleep quality:

Chamomile Tea
Benefits: Chamomile has mild sedative effects and can reduce anxiety and improve sleep quality.
How to Use: Drink a cup of chamomile tea 30-60 minutes before bedtime to help calm the mind.

Valerian Root
Benefits: Valerian root has been used to alleviate anxiety and improve sleep by increasing levels of gamma-aminobutyric acid (GABA), a neurotransmitter that promotes relaxation.
How to Use: Take a valerian root supplement or drink valerian tea an hour before bed. Start with a low dose to assess your tolerance.

Lavender
Benefits: Lavender has calming effects that can reduce anxiety and improve sleep quality.
How to Use: Use a few drops of lavender essential oil in a diffuser before bed, add it to a warm bath, or spray it on your pillow. You can also drink lavender tea or take lavender capsules.

Passionflower
Benefits: Passionflower can reduce anxiety and improve sleep by increasing GABA levels, helping the brain relax.

How to Use: Take a passionflower supplement or drink passionflower tea about 30 minutes before bedtime.

Magnesium

Benefits: Magnesium plays a key role in relaxing muscles and calming the nervous system, which can help relieve anxiety and promote better sleep.

Sources: Dark leafy greens, almonds, pumpkin seeds, and supplements.

How to Use: Take 200-400 mg of magnesium (preferably magnesium glycinate or magnesium citrate) before bed. Consult a doctor to determine the best dose for you.

Cognitive Behavioral Therapy for Insomnia (CBT-I)

Benefits: CBT-I is a therapeutic approach that helps address negative thoughts and behaviors around sleep, reducing anxiety and improving sleep quality.

How to Use: Work with a licensed therapist who specializes in CBT-I. Techniques include relaxation exercises, sleep scheduling, and developing healthy sleep habits.

Exercise and Physical Activity

Benefits: Regular exercise helps reduce anxiety by releasing endorphins and can improve sleep by helping you feel physically tired and relaxed.

How to Use: Aim for at least 30 minutes of moderate exercise most days, but avoid intense workouts close to bedtime as they can be stimulating.

Meditation and Mindfulness

Benefits: Meditation helps calm the mind, reduce stress, and promote relaxation, making it easier to fall asleep.

How to Use: Practice mindfulness meditation daily or try guided meditation apps designed for sleep. Even 5-10 minutes can make a difference in relaxation and anxiety levels.

Deep Breathing Exercises

Benefits: Deep breathing can activate the body's relaxation response, reducing stress and preparing the mind for sleep.

How to Use: Practice deep breathing exercises, such as the 4-7-8 technique (inhale for 4 seconds, hold for 7, and exhale for 8), before bed.

Limit Caffeine and Alcohol

Benefits: Caffeine can increase anxiety and make it harder to fall asleep, while alcohol may disrupt sleep quality and cause awakenings during the night.

How to Use: Avoid caffeine after early afternoon, and limit alcohol in the evening. Opt for herbal teas or water instead.

Warm Baths or Showers

Benefits: A warm bath or shower can help relax muscles and lower the body's core temperature, signaling the body to prepare for sleep.

How to Use: Take a warm bath or shower about an hour before bedtime. Consider adding Epsom salts for extra relaxation.

Ashwagandha

Benefits: Ashwagandha is an adaptogenic herb known for reducing stress and anxiety, helping the body adapt to stressors.

How to Use: Take an ashwagandha supplement (typically 300-600 mg per day) after consulting a healthcare provider.

Reduce Blue Light Exposure Before Bed

Benefits: Blue light from screens can disrupt melatonin production, making it harder to fall asleep.

How to Use: Limit screen use 1-2 hours before bed or use blue light filters. Consider reading a book or engaging in relaxing activities instead.

Progressive Muscle Relaxation (PMR)

Benefits: PMR involves tensing and relaxing different muscle groups, which can help release physical tension and reduce anxiety.

How to Use: Start at your feet and work your way up, tensing each muscle group for a few seconds, then relaxing them.

Journaling

Benefits: Writing down your thoughts can help you release worries, organize thoughts, and create a sense of calm before sleep.

How to Use: Spend a few minutes before bed writing down any worries or to-dos, or keep a gratitude journal to focus on positive aspects of the day.

Healthy Sleep Environment

Benefits: A calm, comfortable sleep environment supports relaxation and better sleep.

How to Use: Keep your bedroom cool, quiet, and dark. Consider blackout curtains, white noise machines, and investing in a comfortable mattress and pillows.

L-Theanine

Benefits: L-theanine is an amino acid found in tea that promotes relaxation without causing drowsiness.

How to Use: L-theanine is available in supplement form, often in doses of 200 mg. Consult with a healthcare provider before use.

Set a Regular Sleep Schedule

Benefits: Going to bed and waking up at the same time each day helps regulate your body's internal clock, improving both sleep quality and reducing anxiety.

How to Use: Aim to go to bed and wake up at the same time every day, even on weekends.

Limit Sugar Intake

Benefits: High sugar intake can cause energy spikes and crashes, worsening anxiety and disrupting sleep.

How to Use: Try to reduce added sugars in your diet by choosing whole foods, fruits, and balanced meals to stabilize blood sugar.

Kava Root

Benefits: Kava root is known for its calming effects and can reduce anxiety, though it should be used with caution due to potential side effects.

How to Use: Take kava root supplements as directed, and consult with a healthcare provider before use, as it can interact with certain medications.

Tips for Managing Anxiety and Improving Sleep Quality

Practice Relaxation Techniques: Techniques like visualization, mindfulness, and guided imagery can prepare the mind and body for rest.

Avoid Napping Late in the Day: While short naps can be beneficial, long or late naps can disrupt nighttime sleep.

Eat a Light Snack if Needed: Avoid heavy meals close to bedtime, but a small snack rich in tryptophan, like yogurt or a banana, can promote sleep.

Limit Fluid Intake Before Bed: Reducing liquids in the evening can help prevent waking up to use the restroom.

Incorporating these natural remedies and lifestyle changes can help reduce anxiety and improve sleep quality. Always consult with a healthcare provider if anxiety or sleep problems persist, as these could be symptoms of underlying health issues.

CHAPTER 7
Skin Health and Beauty

Maintaining healthy, radiant skin is influenced by factors including diet, hydration, lifestyle, and skincare practices. While skincare products are helpful, natural remedies and a holistic approach can also play an important role in achieving glowing, healthy skin. Here are some effective natural remedies and lifestyle tips for promoting skin health and beauty:

Hydration and Drinking Water

Benefits: Staying well-hydrated helps flush out toxins, keeps skin plump, and reduces dryness.

How to Use: Aim for at least 8 glasses of water daily, and increase your intake if you live in a hot climate, exercise frequently, or have dry skin.

Aloe Vera

Benefits: Aloe vera has anti-inflammatory, soothing, and moisturizing properties that help calm the skin, reduce redness, and heal minor burns and acne.

How to Use: Apply fresh aloe vera gel directly to the skin or use products containing pure aloe. Leave it on for 10-15 minutes and rinse with lukewarm water.

Honey

Benefits: Honey is a natural humectant, drawing moisture into the skin. It also has antibacterial properties, making it effective for acne-prone skin.

How to Use: Apply a thin layer of raw honey to your face, leave it on for 15-20 minutes, then rinse with warm water. This can be done 1-2 times a week.

Green Tea

Benefits: Green tea is rich in antioxidants, which help protect the skin from aging and sun damage.

How to Use: Drink 1-2 cups of green tea daily, or apply cooled green tea bags to the skin to reduce puffiness and refresh the complexion. Green tea can also be found in skincare products.

Coconut Oil

Benefits: Coconut oil is highly moisturizing and contains fatty acids that help nourish and repair dry or damaged skin.

How to Use: Apply a small amount of virgin coconut oil to clean skin as a moisturizer, or use it as a makeup remover. Avoid using on acne-prone areas, as it can be comedogenic for some skin types.

Turmeric

Benefits: Turmeric has anti-inflammatory and antioxidant properties that can brighten the skin, reduce hyperpigmentation, and soothe irritation.

How to Use: Mix 1/4 teaspoon of turmeric powder with yogurt or honey to form a paste, apply to the skin for 10-15 minutes, and rinse off. Use caution, as turmeric can stain the skin if left on too long.

Avocado

Benefits: Avocado is rich in healthy fats and vitamins E and C, which help moisturize the skin and support collagen production.

How to Use: Mash up ripe avocado and apply as a mask, leaving it on for 10-15 minutes before rinsing. You can also add avocado oil to your daily skincare routine.

Rose Water

Benefits: Rose water helps balance the skin's pH, reduces redness, and provides a refreshing boost for dull skin.

How to Use: Spray rose water onto the face as a toner or use it throughout the day to refresh your skin. It's also great for setting makeup.

Oatmeal

Benefits: Oatmeal is gentle, soothing, and great for calming irritated or dry skin. It also helps exfoliate and moisturize.

How to Use: Mix oatmeal with warm water or milk to make a paste, apply it to the skin, and leave for 10-15 minutes. This can be especially helpful for eczema-prone skin.

Jojoba Oil

Benefits: Jojoba oil is similar to the skin's natural oils, making it excellent for hydration and balancing oily skin.

How to Use: Apply a few drops of jojoba oil to your face after cleansing as a moisturizer. It's lightweight and non-comedogenic, so it's suitable for most skin types.

Apple Cider Vinegar (ACV)

Benefits: ACV helps balance the skin's pH, reduce bacteria, and may help with acne and blemishes.

How to Use: Dilute ACV with equal parts water and use as a toner, applying with a cotton ball. Start with small amounts to avoid irritation, and avoid using on broken skin.

Healthy Diet for Glowing Skin

Benefits: Eating nutrient-rich foods supports skin health from the inside out, giving your skin the essential vitamins and minerals it needs.

Key Foods: Incorporate leafy greens, berries, nuts, seeds, fatty fish, and foods rich in vitamins A, C, and E. Avoid processed and sugary foods, which can trigger inflammation and breakouts.

Exfoliation with Sugar and Olive Oil

Benefits: Exfoliating removes dead skin cells, allowing fresh skin to emerge and helping prevent clogged pores.
How to Use: Mix sugar with olive oil to create a natural scrub. Gently massage into damp skin, then rinse off. Limit exfoliation to 1-2 times per week to avoid over-exfoliating.

Sunscreen

Benefits: Sunscreen protects the skin from harmful UV rays, preventing sunburn, dark spots, and premature aging.
How to Use: Use a broad-spectrum sunscreen with SPF 30 or higher every day, even on cloudy days, and reapply every 2 hours when outdoors.

Tea Tree Oil for Acne

Benefits: Tea tree oil has antibacterial properties that can help treat and prevent acne without drying out the skin.
How to Use: Dilute tea tree oil with a carrier oil (such as jojoba or coconut oil) before applying it to pimples or acne-prone areas. Avoid using undiluted tea tree oil on sensitive skin.

Cucumber

Benefits: Cucumber is hydrating and has anti-inflammatory properties, making it great for soothing puffiness and irritation.
How to Use: Place chilled cucumber slices on the eyes or blend cucumber and apply it as a face mask to refresh and tone the skin.

Sleep and Stress Management

Benefits: Quality sleep and low-stress levels promote skin repair and reduce signs of aging, while stress can lead to breakouts and dullness.
How to Use: Aim for 7-9 hours of sleep per night and practice stress management techniques like meditation, deep breathing, or yoga to keep your skin looking vibrant.

Vitamin C Serum
Benefits: Vitamin C boosts collagen production, brightens skin tone, and reduces signs of sun damage.
How to Use: Apply a vitamin C serum to clean skin in the morning before moisturizing and applying sunscreen.

Regular Facial Massage
Benefits: Facial massage improves circulation, promoting a healthy glow and reducing puffiness.
How to Use: Use gentle, upward strokes with your fingers or a gua sha tool for a few minutes daily, applying a light facial oil for smooth movement.

Yogurt and Lemon Mask
Benefits: Yogurt contains lactic acid for gentle exfoliation, while lemon has vitamin C for brightening.
How to Use: Mix 1 tablespoon of yogurt with a few drops of lemon juice, apply to the face, and leave on for 10 minutes before rinsing. Lemon can make skin more sensitive to sunlight, so only use this mask at night.

Tips for Maintaining Healthy and Glowing Skin
Establish a Consistent Routine: Use gentle, non-irritating products suited for your skin type, and stick to a routine for the best results.
Avoid Touching Your Face: Touching your face can transfer dirt and oil from your hands to your skin, leading to breakouts.
Use Lukewarm Water: Very hot water can strip natural oils and cause dryness. Wash with lukewarm water instead.
Moisturize Daily: Use a moisturizer that suits your skin type to keep your skin hydrated and protect its barrier.
Incorporating these natural remedies and habits into your routine can enhance skin health, giving you a radiant, youthful complexion

CHAPTER 8
Diabetes and Blood Sugar Management

Managing diabetes and blood sugar levels is essential for preventing complications and promoting overall health. While medication and insulin are often prescribed for diabetes, natural remedies and lifestyle changes can support blood sugar regulation, improve insulin sensitivity, and maintain a healthy weight. Below are some effective natural remedies and lifestyle tips for managing diabetes and maintaining healthy blood sugar levels.

Cinnamon

Benefits: Cinnamon may help lower blood sugar by improving insulin sensitivity and slowing the breakdown of carbohydrates in the digestive tract.

How to Use: Add 1/2 teaspoon of ground cinnamon to smoothies, teas, or oatmeal, or sprinkle it on yogurt. Cinnamon supplements are also available but consult with your doctor before use.

Apple Cider Vinegar

Benefits: Apple cider vinegar (ACV) may help improve insulin sensitivity and lower blood sugar levels after meals.

How to Use: Dilute 1-2 tablespoons of ACV in a glass of water and drink before meals. Be cautious with the acidity and always dilute ACV to prevent tooth enamel erosion and digestive discomfort.

Bitter Melon

Benefits: Bitter melon contains compounds that may mimic insulin and help lower blood sugar levels.

How to Use: Drink bitter melon juice, eat cooked bitter melon, or take bitter melon supplements as recommended by a healthcare provider.

Fenugreek Seeds

Benefits: Fenugreek seeds are high in soluble fiber, which can help manage blood sugar levels by slowing down digestion and absorption of carbohydrates.

How to Use: Soak 1-2 tablespoons of fenugreek seeds overnight and consume them in the morning, or add powdered fenugreek to smoothies and meals.

Gymnema Sylvestre

Benefits: Gymnema sylvestre is an herb that has been shown to help lower blood sugar levels by increasing insulin production and improving insulin sensitivity.

How to Use: Gymnema supplements are available, typically in doses of 200-400 mg daily. Consult with a healthcare provider before use.

Aloe Vera

Benefits: Aloe vera may help regulate blood sugar levels by improving insulin sensitivity and reducing inflammation.

How to Use: Drink aloe vera juice (ensure it is 100% pure and not loaded with added sugar) or take aloe supplements as recommended by a healthcare provider.

Turmeric (Curcumin)

Benefits: Curcumin, the active compound in turmeric, has anti-inflammatory and antioxidant properties that can help manage blood sugar levels and improve insulin sensitivity.

How to Use: Add turmeric to meals, drink turmeric tea, or take curcumin supplements (typically 500-1,000 mg daily). Pair with black pepper for better absorption.

Chromium

Benefits: Chromium is a trace mineral that helps enhance the action of insulin and may improve blood sugar control.

How to Use: Chromium supplements are available, usually in doses of 200-1,000 mcg per day. Include chromium-rich foods like broccoli, eggs, and whole grains in your diet.

Moringa
Benefits: Moringa leaves are rich in antioxidants and compounds that may help lower blood sugar levels and reduce the risk of complications associated with diabetes.
How to Use: Moringa can be consumed in powder form, added to smoothies, or taken as supplements. Aim for 1-2 teaspoons of moringa powder daily.

Low-Glycemic Diet
Benefits: A low-glycemic index (GI) diet helps stabilize blood sugar by reducing spikes after meals.
How to Use: Focus on eating whole grains, legumes, vegetables, and fruits with a low glycemic index. Avoid processed and sugary foods. Incorporate more fiber-rich foods, such as oats, quinoa, and leafy greens.

Exercise
Benefits: Regular physical activity improves insulin sensitivity, helps maintain a healthy weight, and lowers blood sugar levels.
How to Use: Aim for at least 150 minutes of moderate aerobic exercise (such as walking, cycling, or swimming) each week, along with strength training exercises twice a week.

Magnesium
Benefits: Magnesium helps regulate blood sugar levels and improves insulin sensitivity.
Sources: Magnesium-rich foods include spinach, almonds, avocado, and bananas. Magnesium supplements are also available (200-400 mg daily). Always consult a doctor before starting supplements.

Berberine

Benefits: Berberine is a plant compound known for its ability to lower blood sugar levels by increasing insulin sensitivity and reducing liver glucose production.

How to Use: Berberine supplements are typically taken in doses of 500 mg, 2-3 times per day. Consult with a healthcare provider before using berberine, as it can interact with other medications.

Ginger

Benefits: Ginger has anti-inflammatory properties and may help lower blood sugar levels and improve insulin sensitivity.

How to Use: Add fresh ginger to teas, smoothies, or meals, or take ginger supplements (typically 500 mg daily) under the guidance of a healthcare provider.

Lemon

Benefits: Lemon is rich in vitamin C and antioxidants, which may help reduce insulin resistance and regulate blood sugar levels.

How to Use: Add fresh lemon juice to water, salads, or meals, or drink lemon-infused water regularly throughout the day.

Flaxseeds

Benefits: Flaxseeds are high in fiber and omega-3 fatty acids, which can help improve blood sugar control and lower cholesterol levels.

How to Use: Ground flaxseeds are easier to digest than whole seeds. Add them to smoothies, yogurt, or oatmeal for an easy way to incorporate them into your diet.

Coconut Oil

Benefits: Coconut oil contains medium-chain triglycerides (MCTs), which may help improve insulin sensitivity and support weight management.
How to Use: Use coconut oil in cooking or add it to smoothies and baked goods. Aim for 1-2 tablespoons per day.

Stress Reduction Techniques
Benefits: Chronic stress can raise blood sugar levels by increasing cortisol. Managing stress is crucial for blood sugar control.
How to Use: Practice stress-reducing techniques such as yoga, meditation, deep breathing, or spending time outdoors to lower stress and improve blood sugar control.

Balanced Sleep Patterns
Benefits: Poor sleep can lead to insulin resistance and increased blood sugar levels. Getting adequate sleep is important for managing diabetes.
How to Use: Aim for 7-9 hours of sleep each night, establish a consistent bedtime routine, and create a comfortable sleep environment.

Bitter Gourd and Green Tea
Benefits: A combination of bitter gourd and green tea has been shown to reduce blood sugar levels and improve insulin sensitivity.
How to Use: Drink a cup of unsweetened green tea and combine it with bitter gourd juice or cooked bitter gourd for a blood sugar-lowering effect.

Tips for Managing Diabetes and Blood Sugar Levels
Monitor Blood Sugar Levels: Regularly check your blood sugar to track your progress and make necessary adjustments to your diet and lifestyle.
Eat Smaller, More Frequent Meals: Eating balanced meals every 3-4 hours helps maintain steady blood sugar levels.

Avoid Sugary Drinks: Soda, sweetened beverages, and fruit juices can cause rapid blood sugar spikes. Opt for water, herbal teas, or unsweetened beverages instead.
Incorporate Fiber: High-fiber foods help regulate blood sugar by slowing digestion and preventing blood sugar spikes after meals.

By integrating these natural remedies, dietary changes, and lifestyle habits, you can better manage your blood sugar levels and overall health. Always consult your healthcare provider before making significant changes to your treatment plan or starting new supplements, especially if you're on medications for diabetes.

CHAPTER 9

Allergy Relief

Allergies can cause a wide range of symptoms, from mild irritation like sneezing and itchy eyes to more severe reactions such as difficulty breathing. While traditional treatments like antihistamines and decongestants are commonly used, there are several natural remedies that can help alleviate allergy symptoms and support your immune system. Below are some natural methods for managing allergies:

Local Honey

Benefits: Local honey may help build immunity to local pollen and reduce seasonal allergy symptoms.

How to Use: Consume a teaspoon of local honey daily to potentially help your body build a tolerance to allergens. This is best done starting a few months before allergy season begins.

Apple Cider Vinegar

Benefits: Apple cider vinegar is believed to help clear mucus, reduce inflammation, and detoxify the body, easing symptoms like nasal congestion and sinus pressure.

How to Use: Dilute 1-2 tablespoons of apple cider vinegar in a glass of water and drink 1-2 times per day. You can also gargle with it to soothe a sore throat caused by allergies.

Neti Pot (Saline Nasal Irrigation)

Benefits: Nasal irrigation helps rinse out allergens like pollen, dust, and mold from the nasal passages, providing immediate relief from congestion and sinus pressure.

How to Use: Use a neti pot with a saline solution to irrigate your nasal passages once or twice a day, especially during allergy season. Make sure to use distilled or boiled water that has been cooled to avoid infections.

Butterbur

Benefits: Butterbur is an herb that has been found to help alleviate hay fever and seasonal allergy symptoms by reducing histamine release and inflammation.

How to Use: Butterbur supplements (around 50-75 mg, twice daily) can be taken as directed. Choose products that are free of pyrrolizidine alkaloids (PA), which can be toxic to the liver.

Quercetin

Benefits: Quercetin is a flavonoid found in many fruits, vegetables, and grains. It has natural antihistamine properties and can help stabilize mast cells to prevent the release of histamine.

How to Use: Quercetin supplements are available (typically 500 mg, 1-2 times daily). It's also found in foods like apples, onions, and berries, so eating these regularly can provide a natural boost.

Probiotics

Benefits: Probiotics help balance gut bacteria, which plays a key role in immune system function. A healthy gut microbiome can help regulate allergic responses and reduce inflammation.

How to Use: Take a high-quality probiotic supplement daily, or eat probiotic-rich foods like yogurt, kefir, sauerkraut, kimchi, and kombucha to support your immune health.

Essential Oils

Benefits: Certain essential oils can help alleviate allergy symptoms by clearing nasal congestion, reducing inflammation, and promoting relaxation.

How to Use:

Peppermint Oil: Apply diluted peppermint oil (mixed with a carrier oil) to the chest or under the nose to help open nasal passages.
Lavender Oil: Lavender has antihistamine properties and can help reduce sneezing and itching. Use it in a diffuser, or dilute it and apply to the temples or wrists.
Eucalyptus Oil: Eucalyptus helps reduce inflammation and acts as a natural decongestant. Use it in a steam inhalation, or diffuse it in the air.

Stinging Nettle

Benefits: Stinging nettle is a natural antihistamine and may help relieve symptoms of hay fever, including sneezing, itchy eyes, and congestion.
How to Use: Stinging nettle supplements (typically 300-500 mg, 2-3 times per day) can be taken during allergy season, or you can brew nettle tea to drink.

Vitamin C

Benefits: Vitamin C is a powerful antioxidant that can help boost the immune system and reduce the release of histamine, which contributes to allergy symptoms.
How to Use: Aim for 500-1,000 mg of vitamin C daily. You can also consume vitamin C-rich foods such as oranges, strawberries, kiwi, bell peppers, and leafy greens.

Echinacea

Benefits: Echinacea is an herb that may help strengthen the immune system and reduce inflammation, which is beneficial for allergy sufferers.
How to Use: Echinacea can be taken as a tea or in supplement form (typically 300 mg, 3 times a day). It may help reduce symptoms like sinus congestion and itchy throat.

Garlic

Benefits: Garlic has anti-inflammatory properties and may help reduce allergic reactions by boosting the immune system.

How to Use: Add fresh garlic to meals, or take garlic supplements (usually 300-500 mg, 2-3 times per day) to help manage allergy symptoms.

Turmeric

Benefits: Turmeric contains curcumin, a compound with potent anti-inflammatory and antioxidant properties that can help alleviate allergy symptoms such as nasal congestion and inflammation.

How to Use: Add turmeric to your diet or drink turmeric tea. You can also take turmeric supplements (500-1,000 mg, 1-2 times a day) to reduce symptoms.

Saltwater Gargle

Benefits: Gargling with warm saltwater can help soothe a sore throat caused by post-nasal drip and reduce inflammation.

How to Use: Mix 1/2 teaspoon of salt in a glass of warm water, gargle for 30 seconds, and repeat several times a day as needed.

Hydration

Benefits: Staying hydrated helps thin mucus, making it easier to clear allergens from the body. Proper hydration also helps reduce nasal congestion and dryness.

How to Use: Drink plenty of water throughout the day to help keep mucus thin and relieve allergy symptoms. Herbal teas like ginger or peppermint tea can also be helpful.

Avoiding Triggers

Benefits: Reducing exposure to allergens like pollen, dust, and pet dander is key to preventing allergy flare-ups.

How to Use:
Indoors: Keep windows closed during high pollen seasons, use air purifiers, and wash bedding frequently to reduce dust mites and pet dander.
Outdoors: Limit outdoor activities when pollen counts are high, wear sunglasses to protect your eyes, and wash your hands and face after being outside.

Lifestyle Tips for Managing Allergies
Keep your home clean: Regularly clean and vacuum using a HEPA filter, and wash bedding in hot water to remove allergens.
Use an air purifier: Invest in a HEPA air purifier for your home, especially in the bedroom, to help filter out airborne allergens.
Wear a mask: When working outside during allergy season, wear a mask to reduce exposure to pollen and other allergens.
Shower before bed: Shower and change clothes before bed to remove allergens that may have settled on your skin and hair throughout the day.

Natural remedies, such as herbal supplements, essential oils, and dietary changes, can complement conventional treatments for allergies, providing relief from symptoms and improving overall immune function. As with any treatment, it's important to consult a healthcare provider before using new remedies, especially if you have a history of severe allergic reactions or are taking medications.

CHAPTER 10
Cholesterol Management

Managing cholesterol levels is essential for maintaining heart health and reducing the risk of cardiovascular diseases, such as heart attacks and strokes. While medications like statins are commonly prescribed, there are several natural remedies and lifestyle changes that can help regulate cholesterol levels. Below are some natural strategies for managing cholesterol levels.

Soluble Fiber

Benefits: Soluble fiber helps lower LDL (bad) cholesterol by binding to cholesterol in the digestive system and preventing its absorption into the bloodstream.

Sources: Foods high in soluble fiber include oats, barley, beans, lentils, apples, pears, and carrots.

How to Use: Aim to include at least 25-30 grams of fiber in your daily diet. Breakfast oatmeal, salads with beans, or smoothies with fruits and vegetables are great ways to boost fiber intake.

Omega-3 Fatty Acids

Benefits: Omega-3 fatty acids help lower triglycerides, reduce inflammation, and improve overall heart health by raising HDL (good) cholesterol and lowering LDL (bad) cholesterol.

Sources: Fatty fish (like salmon, mackerel, sardines), chia seeds, flaxseeds, walnuts, and omega-3 supplements.

How to Use: Aim for at least two servings of fatty fish per week or take omega-3 supplements (typically 1,000-2,000 mg daily). Ground flaxseeds and chia seeds can be added to smoothies or oatmeal for an additional boost.

Plant Sterols and Stanols

Benefits: Plant sterols and stanols are compounds found in plants that can help lower LDL cholesterol by blocking cholesterol absorption in the intestines.

Sources: Foods fortified with plant sterols, such as certain margarines, yogurt drinks, and fruit juices, as well as nuts, seeds, and whole grains.

How to Use: Aim for 1-2 grams of plant sterols and stanols per day. Look for fortified food products or take supplements as advised by a healthcare provider.

Garlic

Benefits: Garlic has been shown to help reduce total cholesterol, LDL cholesterol, and triglycerides, while also improving overall heart health.

How to Use: Eat 1-2 raw garlic cloves per day, or take garlic supplements (typically 600-1,200 mg daily). You can also add garlic to meals like soups, salads, and roasted vegetables.

Turmeric (Curcumin)

Benefits: Curcumin, the active compound in turmeric, has anti-inflammatory properties and has been shown to help lower cholesterol levels and improve overall heart health.

How to Use: Add turmeric to meals or drink turmeric tea. You can also take curcumin supplements (typically 500-1,000 mg daily) with black pepper for better absorption.

Green Tea

Benefits: Green tea contains catechins, antioxidants that can help lower LDL cholesterol and triglycerides, and support heart health.

How to Use: Drink 2-3 cups of green tea daily, or take green tea extract supplements (typically 250-500 mg per day). Choose unsweetened green tea for maximum benefits.

Red Yeast Rice

Benefits: Red yeast rice contains natural statins that may help lower LDL cholesterol levels and improve overall heart health.

How to Use: Red yeast rice supplements are available (typically 600-1,200 mg per day). Consult with a healthcare provider before use, especially if you are already taking statins.

Coenzyme Q10 (CoQ10)

Benefits: CoQ10 is an antioxidant that helps improve heart health and may be beneficial for individuals taking statin medications, which can deplete CoQ10 levels.

How to Use: CoQ10 supplements (typically 100-200 mg daily) can be taken to support heart health and combat side effects from statin use.

Olive Oil

Benefits: Olive oil, especially extra virgin olive oil, is high in monounsaturated fats, which can help increase HDL cholesterol and lower LDL cholesterol.

How to Use: Use olive oil as your primary cooking oil or drizzle it over salads and vegetables. Aim for about 2 tablespoons per day for heart health benefits.

Nuts (Almonds, Walnuts, Pistachios)

Benefits: Nuts are rich in healthy fats, fiber, and antioxidants, and have been shown to help lower LDL cholesterol and improve heart health.

How to Use: A handful of unsalted nuts (about 1 ounce) per day is sufficient for heart health. Almonds, walnuts, and pistachios are especially beneficial.

Avocado

Benefits: Avocados are a good source of monounsaturated fats and fiber, which can help lower LDL cholesterol and raise HDL cholesterol.

How to Use: Add 1/2 to 1 avocado to salads, sandwiches, or smoothies daily to benefit from its cholesterol-lowering properties.

Cinnamon

Benefits: Cinnamon contains antioxidants that can help lower total cholesterol, LDL cholesterol, and triglycerides, while also supporting heart health.

How to Use: Add 1/2 teaspoon of cinnamon to oatmeal, smoothies, or yogurt, or sprinkle it on your coffee or tea. Cinnamon supplements are also available but consult a healthcare provider before use.

Exercise

Benefits: Regular physical activity helps increase HDL cholesterol and decrease LDL cholesterol and triglycerides, improving overall cardiovascular health.

How to Use: Aim for at least 150 minutes of moderate aerobic exercise (like walking, cycling, or swimming) per week, along with strength training exercises twice a week.

Maintain a Healthy Weight

Benefits: Losing excess weight, especially belly fat, can help lower LDL cholesterol and triglycerides while increasing HDL cholesterol.

How to Use: Focus on a balanced, nutrient-rich diet and regular exercise to achieve and maintain a healthy weight.

Limit Saturated and Trans Fats

Benefits: Saturated and trans fats can raise LDL cholesterol levels and contribute to heart disease.

How to Use: Avoid foods high in trans fats (such as fried foods, processed snacks, and baked goods) and limit saturated fats found in red meat, full-fat dairy products, and processed meats.

Avoid Added Sugars and Refined Carbs
Benefits: Diets high in added sugars and refined carbohydrates can lead to higher triglyceride levels and lower HDL cholesterol, increasing the risk of cardiovascular disease.
How to Use: Limit processed foods, sugary drinks, and refined grains, and focus on whole grains, vegetables, and fruits in your diet.

Flaxseeds
Benefits: Flaxseeds are rich in fiber and omega-3 fatty acids, both of which can help lower LDL cholesterol and triglycerides.
How to Use: Add ground flaxseeds to smoothies, oatmeal, or yogurt, or sprinkle them on salads. Aim for 1-2 tablespoons per day.
18. Soy Protein
Benefits: Soy protein has been shown to reduce LDL cholesterol levels and improve overall heart health.
Sources: Foods like tofu, tempeh, soy milk, and edamame are good sources of soy protein.
How to Use: Include 1-2 servings of soy-based foods in your diet daily to help manage cholesterol levels.

Lifestyle Tips for Cholesterol Management
Monitor Your Cholesterol Levels: Regular cholesterol testing is important to track your progress and make adjustments to your diet and lifestyle.
Quit Smoking: Smoking lowers HDL cholesterol and contributes to the buildup of plaque in arteries, increasing the risk of cardiovascular disease.
Limit Alcohol Consumption: Excessive alcohol intake can raise triglycerides and contribute to other heart health issues. Limit alcohol to one drink per day for women and two drinks per day for men.

Stay Hydrated: Drink plenty of water throughout the day to maintain proper metabolic function and support overall health.

Managing cholesterol naturally involves a combination of diet, exercise, and lifestyle changes. By incorporating heart-healthy foods, supplements, and habits into your routine, you can improve your cholesterol levels and reduce the risk of heart disease. Always consult with a healthcare provider before making significant changes to your diet or taking new supplements, especially if you have an existing heart condition or are on medication for cholesterol.

CHAPTER 11

Weight Loss and Metabolism Boosters

Maintaining a healthy weight is essential for overall well-being and can significantly reduce the risk of developing chronic conditions like diabetes, heart disease, and high blood pressure. In addition to a balanced diet and regular exercise, there are several natural remedies and lifestyle changes that can help boost metabolism and promote weight loss. Below are some effective strategies:

Green Tea and Green Tea Extract

Benefits: Green tea contains catechins, particularly epigallocatechin gallate (EGCG), which have been shown to boost metabolism and enhance fat burning.

How to Use: Drink 2-3 cups of green tea daily, or take green tea extract supplements (typically 250-500 mg per day) to support fat loss. Choose unsweetened green tea for best results.

Apple Cider Vinegar

Benefits: Apple cider vinegar (ACV) can help control blood sugar levels and promote feelings of fullness, leading to reduced calorie intake. It also has the potential to boost metabolism slightly.

How to Use: Mix 1-2 tablespoons of ACV with a glass of water and drink before meals to help reduce appetite and improve digestion. Start with smaller amounts to avoid digestive discomfort.

Cayenne Pepper (Capsaicin)

Benefits: The active compound in cayenne pepper, capsaicin, has been shown to increase metabolism and promote fat burning by raising body temperature and increasing calorie expenditure.

How to Use: Add cayenne pepper to meals, or take cayenne pepper supplements (typically 500-1,000 mg per day). Start with small amounts, as it can be quite spicy for some individuals.

Ginger

Benefits: Ginger is known to have thermogenic properties, which can help increase metabolism and promote fat burning. It also aids digestion and can reduce bloating.

How to Use: Add fresh ginger to smoothies, teas, or stir-fries, or drink ginger tea regularly. You can also take ginger supplements (typically 500-1,000 mg per day).

Lemon Water

Benefits: Drinking water infused with lemon can help improve metabolism by boosting hydration and promoting digestion. The vitamin C in lemons may also help with fat oxidation.

How to Use: Squeeze the juice of half a lemon into a glass of warm or cold water and drink it first thing in the morning or before meals to help promote fat loss.

Protein-Rich Foods

Benefits: Protein has a high thermic effect, meaning it requires more energy to digest than fats or carbohydrates, thus boosting metabolism. Protein also helps promote feelings of fullness, reducing overall calorie intake.

Sources: Lean meats, fish, eggs, legumes, tofu, and Greek yogurt are excellent sources of protein.

How to Use: Include a source of protein in every meal and snack to support weight loss and boost metabolism. Aim for 20-30 grams of protein per meal.

Coconut Oil

Benefits: Coconut oil contains medium-chain triglycerides (MCTs), which are metabolized differently than other fats and can increase calorie burning.

How to Use: Use coconut oil for cooking or add it to smoothies and coffee. Aim for 1-2 tablespoons per day for weight loss benefits.

Coffee (Caffeine)

Benefits: Caffeine is a natural stimulant that can increase metabolism and promote fat burning by enhancing fat mobilization. It also increases alertness and energy levels.

How to Use: Drink 1-2 cups of black coffee or consume caffeine-containing beverages like green tea or yerba mate to boost metabolism. Avoid excess caffeine, as it can cause jitteriness or digestive discomfort.

Intermittent Fasting

Benefits: Intermittent fasting is an eating pattern that involves alternating periods of eating and fasting. It may help boost metabolism, improve fat burning, and increase insulin sensitivity, which aids in weight loss.

How to Use: There are several approaches to intermittent fasting, such as the 16/8 method (fasting for 16 hours and eating within an 8-hour window), or the 5:2 method (eating normally for 5 days and restricting calories on 2 non-consecutive days). Choose an approach that suits your lifestyle.

High-Intensity Interval Training (HIIT)

Benefits: HIIT is an exercise regimen that alternates between short bursts of intense activity and rest periods. It has been shown to boost metabolism and promote fat burning, even after the workout is over.

How to Use: Incorporate HIIT into your workout routine 2-3 times per week. It can be done with activities like sprinting, cycling, or bodyweight exercises such as squats and push-ups.

Drink More Water

Benefits: Staying hydrated is crucial for optimal metabolic function. Drinking water before meals can also help reduce appetite and prevent overeating.

How to Use: Aim to drink at least 8 cups (64 ounces) of water per day, and consider drinking a glass of water 30 minutes before meals to help control hunger.

Sleep and Stress Management

Benefits: Poor sleep and chronic stress can disrupt metabolism and increase hunger hormones, leading to overeating and weight gain. Managing stress and getting enough quality sleep are essential for weight loss.

How to Use: Aim for 7-9 hours of sleep per night and incorporate stress management techniques like meditation, deep breathing exercises, or yoga to maintain a healthy metabolism.

MCT Oil

Benefits: MCT oil, derived from coconut oil, contains medium-chain triglycerides that are metabolized quickly by the liver and used as an energy source, increasing fat burning.

How to Use: Add 1 tablespoon of MCT oil to smoothies, coffee, or salad dressings to support metabolism and enhance energy levels. Start with smaller amounts to avoid digestive discomfort.

Apple Cider Vinegar (ACV)

Benefits: ACV helps regulate blood sugar levels and increase feelings of fullness, which can help with weight loss. It also aids in digestion.

How to Use: Mix 1-2 tablespoons of ACV with water and drink it before meals. You can also add it to salad dressings or marinades.

Fiber-Rich Foods

Benefits: Foods high in fiber slow down digestion, helping you feel full longer and preventing overeating. Fiber also supports a healthy gut, which plays a role in metabolism.
Sources: Whole grains, beans, fruits, vegetables, and legumes are excellent sources of fiber.
How to Use: Aim for at least 25-30 grams of fiber per day from a variety of whole, plant-based foods.

Dandelion Tea

Benefits: Dandelion has natural diuretic properties, helping the body expel excess water weight. It also supports liver function and digestion.
How to Use: Drink 1-2 cups of dandelion tea daily, especially if you are looking to reduce water retention.

Fiber Supplements (Psyllium Husk)

Benefits: Psyllium husk is a natural fiber supplement that helps with digestion and promotes feelings of fullness, which can lead to reduced calorie intake.
How to Use: Take 1-2 teaspoons of psyllium husk with a large glass of water before meals to help manage appetite and improve digestion.

Healthy Fats

Benefits: Healthy fats, such as those found in avocados, nuts, seeds, and olive oil, help increase satiety and regulate blood sugar levels, which supports weight loss.
How to Use: Include moderate amounts of healthy fats in your diet to promote feelings of fullness and prevent overeating.

There are many natural remedies and lifestyle changes that can help boost metabolism and promote weight loss. These strategies can be effective when combined with a balanced diet, regular physical activity, and adequate sleep. As always, it's important to consult a healthcare provider before starting any new supplement or weight loss program, especially if you have underlying health conditions.

CHAPTER 12
Natural Remedies for Women's Health

Women's health encompasses a wide range of concerns, from hormonal imbalances and menstrual issues to menopause, fertility, and bone health. Many natural remedies and lifestyle changes can help support women's well-being at every stage of life. Below are some effective natural remedies for common women's health issues:

Hormonal Balance

Herbs for Hormonal Balance:

Chaste Tree (Vitex): This herb is known to help regulate menstrual cycles and alleviate symptoms of premenstrual syndrome (PMS) and hormonal imbalances.

How to Use: Take chaste tree supplements (typically 400-800 mg daily) or drink it as a tea to help balance hormones.

Maca Root: Maca root is another herb that may help regulate hormones, improve energy levels, and reduce symptoms of menopause and PMS.

How to Use: Maca root can be consumed in powder form (1-3 teaspoons daily) or as a supplement.

Menstrual Pain Relief

Ginger and Turmeric:

Benefits: Both ginger and turmeric have anti-inflammatory properties that may help reduce menstrual cramps and relieve pain.

How to Use: Drink ginger or turmeric tea during your period, or take supplements (500-1,000 mg daily) to ease cramps.

Essential Oils:

Benefits: Essential oils like lavender, clary sage, and peppermint have soothing properties that can help reduce menstrual discomfort.

How to Use: Dilute a few drops of essential oils in a carrier oil (like coconut oil) and massage into the lower abdomen to relieve cramps.

Menopause Support
Black Cohosh:
Benefits: Black cohosh is often used to alleviate symptoms of menopause, including hot flashes, mood swings, and night sweats.
How to Use: Take black cohosh supplements (typically 40-80 mg daily) or drink black cohosh tea.
Red Clover:
Benefits: Red clover contains isoflavones, which are plant-based compounds that mimic estrogen and may help balance hormones during menopause.
How to Use: Drink red clover tea (1-2 cups daily) or take red clover supplements (typically 40-80 mg daily).

Bone Health
Calcium and Vitamin D:
Benefits: Calcium and vitamin D are essential for maintaining strong bones and preventing osteoporosis. They help regulate bone mineral density and support overall bone health.
How to Use: Include calcium-rich foods like leafy greens, dairy, and fortified plant milks in your diet. Consider taking a calcium and vitamin D supplement if you are not getting enough from food sources.
Magnesium:
Benefits: Magnesium helps with calcium absorption and bone mineralization, supporting bone health and preventing bone loss.
How to Use: Eat magnesium-rich foods like almonds, spinach, and avocados, or take magnesium supplements (typically 200-400 mg daily).

Fertility Support

Raspberry Leaf:

Benefits: Raspberry leaf is often used to tone the uterus and regulate menstrual cycles, potentially improving fertility. It's especially beneficial for women trying to conceive.

How to Use: Drink 1-2 cups of raspberry leaf tea daily to support reproductive health and balance hormones.

Vitex (Chaste Tree):

Benefits: Vitex is commonly used to balance hormones and regulate menstrual cycles, which can improve fertility.

How to Use: Take Vitex supplements (typically 400-800 mg daily) for several months to improve ovulation and fertility.

Urinary Tract Health

Cranberry:

Benefits: Cranberry is well-known for its ability to prevent urinary tract infections (UTIs) by preventing bacteria from adhering to the urinary tract walls.

How to Use: Drink unsweetened cranberry juice or take cranberry supplements (typically 500 mg-1,000 mg daily).

D-Mannose:

Benefits: D-Mannose is a sugar that can prevent bacteria from sticking to the urinary tract, helping to reduce the risk of UTIs.

How to Use: Take D-Mannose supplements (typically 500-1,000 mg daily) as a preventive measure.

Skin Health

Aloe Vera:

Benefits: Aloe vera is known for its healing properties and can help treat dry skin, acne, and minor burns.

How to Use: Apply fresh aloe vera gel directly to the skin, or use an aloe-based moisturizer for daily hydration.

Tea Tree Oil:

Benefits: Tea tree oil has antibacterial and anti-inflammatory properties that can help treat acne and skin irritations.

How to Use: Apply diluted tea tree oil (2-3 drops in a carrier oil) directly to blemishes or skin infections.

Mood and Mental Health
St. John's Wort:
Benefits: St. John's Wort is commonly used to help manage symptoms of depression, anxiety, and mild mood disorders.
How to Use: Take St. John's Wort supplements (typically 300 mg 3 times daily), or drink it as a tea.
Ashwagandha:
Benefits: Ashwagandha is an adaptogenic herb that can help reduce stress and anxiety, balance mood, and improve sleep quality.
How to Use: Take ashwagandha supplements (typically 300-600 mg daily) to support mental health and overall well-being.

Digestive Health
Peppermint Tea:
Benefits: Peppermint has soothing properties that can help with indigestion, bloating, and stomach cramps.
How to Use: Drink 1-2 cups of peppermint tea daily to alleviate digestive discomfort.
Probiotics:
Benefits: Probiotics help restore the balance of healthy gut bacteria, which is essential for digestion and immune function.
How to Use: Take probiotic supplements (typically 5-10 billion CFU daily) or consume probiotic-rich foods like yogurt, kefir, sauerkraut, and kimchi.

Breast Health
Flaxseed:
Benefits: Flaxseeds contain lignans, which may help balance hormones and support breast health by acting as phytoestrogens.

How to Use: Add ground flaxseeds to smoothies, oatmeal, or salads. Aim for 1-2 tablespoons daily.
Evening Primrose Oil:
Benefits: Evening primrose oil is rich in gamma-linolenic acid (GLA), which may help alleviate symptoms of fibrocystic breasts and support overall breast health.
How to Use: Take evening primrose oil supplements (typically 500-1,000 mg daily) for breast pain and hormonal balance.

Hair Health
Biotin:
Benefits: Biotin is a B-vitamin that plays a key role in hair health and may help reduce hair thinning.
How to Use: Take biotin supplements (typically 2,500-5,000 mcg daily) or eat biotin-rich foods like eggs, nuts, and leafy greens.
Rosemary Oil:
Benefits: Rosemary oil has been shown to stimulate hair growth by improving circulation to the scalp and promoting hair follicle health.
How to Use: Massage a few drops of diluted rosemary essential oil into the scalp 2-3 times per week to support healthy hair growth.

Natural remedies can offer support for many aspects of women's health, from hormonal balance to fertility and bone health. By incorporating these natural remedies into your routine, you can improve your well-being without relying solely on pharmaceuticals. However, it's important to consult with a healthcare provider before starting any new supplement or remedy, especially if you have underlying health conditions or are pregnant or breastfeeding.

CHAPTER 13
Men's Health and Vitality

Men's health concerns span various issues, including reproductive health, energy levels, muscle strength, cardiovascular health, and mental well-being. While medical interventions can be important, many natural remedies and lifestyle changes can also play a significant role in maintaining vitality and addressing common health challenges. Below are effective natural remedies for supporting men's health and vitality:

Testosterone Support
Fenugreek:
Benefits: Fenugreek is a herb that has been shown to help increase testosterone levels and improve libido. It also helps regulate blood sugar levels.
How to Use: Take fenugreek supplements (typically 500-600 mg daily) or add fenugreek seeds to your diet.
Zinc:
Benefits: Zinc is an essential mineral for testosterone production and male fertility. It supports immune function and plays a key role in maintaining healthy testosterone levels.
How to Use: Consume zinc-rich foods like oysters, pumpkin seeds, and spinach, or take zinc supplements (typically 15-30 mg daily).
Ashwagandha:
Benefits: This adaptogen helps reduce stress, which can support optimal testosterone levels. Ashwagandha is also known for improving strength, stamina, and sexual health.
How to Use: Take ashwagandha supplements (typically 300-500 mg daily) for stress reduction and testosterone support.

Erectile Dysfunction (ED)
L-Arginine:

Benefits: L-arginine is an amino acid that helps improve blood flow by boosting nitric oxide levels. This can help with erectile function and overall cardiovascular health.

How to Use: Take L-arginine supplements (typically 500-1,000 mg daily) or consume foods high in L-arginine, such as nuts, seeds, and lean meats.

Ginseng:

Benefits: Ginseng is known for its ability to improve erectile function and increase libido by enhancing blood flow and reducing fatigue.

How to Use: Take ginseng supplements (typically 200-400 mg daily), or drink ginseng tea to improve sexual health.

Yohimbine:

Benefits: Yohimbine is an herbal supplement that may improve erectile function by enhancing blood flow to the penis.

How to Use: Consult a healthcare provider before using yohimbine, as it can cause side effects such as increased heart rate and anxiety.

Muscle Mass and Strength

Creatine:

Benefits: Creatine is a natural compound found in muscle cells that helps increase muscle mass, strength, and performance during high-intensity workouts.

How to Use: Take creatine monohydrate supplements (typically 3-5 grams daily) to improve strength, energy, and muscle growth.

Whey Protein:

Benefits: Whey protein is an excellent source of high-quality protein that supports muscle repair and growth after exercise.

How to Use: Consume 20-30 grams of whey protein in a shake or smoothie after workouts to enhance muscle recovery and growth.

Heart Health

Omega-3 Fatty Acids:
Benefits: Omega-3 fatty acids, found in fish oil and flaxseeds, are known for their cardiovascular benefits, including reducing inflammation and improving cholesterol levels.
How to Use: Take fish oil supplements (typically 1,000-3,000 mg daily) or include fatty fish (like salmon, mackerel, and sardines) and flaxseeds in your diet.
Coenzyme Q10 (CoQ10):
Benefits: CoQ10 is an antioxidant that helps improve heart health by enhancing energy production in cells and reducing oxidative stress.
How to Use: Take CoQ10 supplements (typically 100-200 mg daily) to support heart health and overall vitality.
Hawthorn Berry:
Benefits: Hawthorn berry is a powerful herb that supports heart health by improving blood flow, lowering blood pressure, and enhancing cardiovascular function.
How to Use: Take hawthorn berry supplements (typically 250-500 mg daily) or drink hawthorn berry tea.

Prostate Health
Saw Palmetto:
Benefits: Saw palmetto is widely used to support prostate health, reduce symptoms of benign prostatic hyperplasia (BPH), and promote urinary function.
How to Use: Take saw palmetto supplements (typically 320 mg daily) to support prostate health and reduce urinary symptoms.
Pumpkin Seeds:
Benefits: Pumpkin seeds are rich in zinc and phytosterols, which are beneficial for prostate health and may help reduce the risk of prostate enlargement.
How to Use: Eat a handful of roasted pumpkin seeds daily or take pumpkin seed oil supplements.

Mental Clarity and Cognitive Function

Ginkgo Biloba:
Benefits: Ginkgo biloba is known for its ability to improve blood circulation to the brain, enhancing memory, focus, and cognitive function.
How to Use: Take ginkgo biloba supplements (typically 120-240 mg daily) to improve mental clarity and brain health.
Rhodiola Rosea:
Benefits: Rhodiola is an adaptogen that helps combat mental fatigue, reduce stress, and improve cognitive performance.
How to Use: Take rhodiola supplements (typically 200-400 mg daily) to support brain health and mental vitality.
Bacopa Monnieri:
Benefits: Bacopa is an herb known for its ability to enhance memory, concentration, and cognitive performance, while also reducing anxiety and stress.
How to Use: Take bacopa supplements (typically 300-450 mg daily) to support cognitive function and mental clarity.

Stress and Anxiety Relief
Ashwagandha:
Benefits: As mentioned earlier, ashwagandha helps reduce stress and anxiety, which can negatively impact overall health and vitality.
How to Use: Take ashwagandha supplements (typically 300-500 mg daily) or drink it as a tea to manage stress and improve mood.
Lavender Oil:
Benefits: Lavender oil is well-known for its calming properties and can help reduce anxiety, improve sleep, and promote relaxation.
How to Use: Diffuse lavender oil in your home, add a few drops to a bath, or massage diluted oil onto your temples for stress relief.

Sleep and Restorative Health
Melatonin:

Benefits: Melatonin is a hormone that regulates the sleep-wake cycle. Supplementing with melatonin can help improve sleep quality and regulate sleep patterns.
How to Use: Take melatonin supplements (typically 1-5 mg) 30-60 minutes before bedtime to support restful sleep.
Magnesium:
Benefits: Magnesium helps relax muscles and promotes better sleep quality by calming the nervous system.
How to Use: Take magnesium supplements (typically 200-400 mg daily) or consume magnesium-rich foods like almonds, spinach, and avocado.
Valerian Root:
Benefits: Valerian root is a natural herb that promotes relaxation and reduces anxiety, improving the ability to fall and stay asleep.
How to Use: Take valerian root supplements (typically 300-600 mg) before bedtime to enhance sleep quality.

Hair Growth and Scalp Health
Saw Palmetto (for Hair Loss):
Benefits: Saw palmetto is believed to reduce the effects of DHT (dihydrotestosterone), a hormone linked to male-pattern baldness.
How to Use: Take saw palmetto supplements (typically 320 mg daily) to support hair growth and prevent hair thinning.
Rosemary Oil:
Benefits: Rosemary oil can improve circulation to the scalp, promoting hair growth and reducing hair loss.
How to Use: Massage diluted rosemary essential oil into the scalp 2-3 times per week to stimulate hair follicles.

Natural remedies can help improve many aspects of men's health, from supporting testosterone and reproductive health to boosting mental clarity, reducing stress, and enhancing physical vitality. These remedies, when combined with a balanced diet, regular exercise, and healthy lifestyle choices, can contribute significantly to maintaining overall well-being and vitality at any age. As always, consult a healthcare provider before starting any new supplement or remedy to ensure it's appropriate for your individual health needs.

CHAPTER 14
Detoxification and Cleansing

Detoxification is the process of eliminating harmful substances from the body, and cleansing focuses on supporting organs such as the liver, kidneys, and digestive system to improve overall health and vitality. While the body has its own detoxifying systems, natural remedies can support and enhance this process, helping to remove toxins, improve energy levels, and promote optimal health.

Below are some effective natural remedies for detoxification and cleansing:

Hydration
Water:
Benefits: Staying hydrated is crucial for detoxification, as water helps flush toxins out through the kidneys and supports the overall function of the liver and digestive system.
How to Use: Drink at least 8 glasses (2 liters) of water daily. Adding lemon, cucumber, or mint can enhance the detoxifying properties of water.
Lemon Water:
Benefits: Lemon contains vitamin C and antioxidants, which can help stimulate the liver, boost the immune system, and support digestion.
How to Use: Start your day with a glass of warm lemon water to stimulate digestion and detoxification.

Liver Support
Milk Thistle:
Benefits: Milk thistle is a well-known herb that supports liver health by promoting detoxification and protecting liver cells from damage. It contains silymarin, an antioxidant that helps the liver regenerate.

How to Use: Take milk thistle supplements (typically 150-300 mg, 2-3 times daily) or drink milk thistle tea to support liver function.

Dandelion Root:

Benefits: Dandelion root is a natural diuretic that helps flush out toxins through the kidneys and supports liver detoxification.

How to Use: Drink dandelion root tea (1-2 cups daily) or take dandelion supplements (typically 500 mg-1,000 mg daily).

Colon Cleansing

Psyllium Husk:

Benefits: Psyllium husk is a natural fiber that helps promote regular bowel movements and eliminate waste and toxins from the digestive system.

How to Use: Take psyllium husk powder (typically 1-2 teaspoons in water, 1-2 times per day) to improve bowel regularity and cleanse the colon.

Aloe Vera:

Benefits: Aloe vera has soothing properties that can help cleanse the colon and improve digestion, while also supporting the body's natural detoxification processes.

How to Use: Drink 1-2 tablespoons of aloe vera juice (unsweetened) daily to support digestion and colon cleansing.

Cleansing Herbal Teas:

Benefits: Teas made from herbs like ginger, peppermint, and senna can help stimulate digestion, relieve bloating, and support the elimination of waste.

How to Use: Drink herbal cleansing teas (such as ginger, peppermint, or senna) 1-2 times daily for gentle colon cleansing.

Kidney Detox

Cranberry Juice:

Benefits: Cranberry juice is known for supporting kidney health and preventing urinary tract infections (UTIs) by helping to flush out harmful bacteria and toxins.

How to Use: Drink unsweetened cranberry juice (1 cup daily) or take cranberry supplements (typically 500 mg daily) to support kidney health and detoxification.

Parsley:

Benefits: Parsley is a natural diuretic that helps cleanse the kidneys and urinary system, promoting the removal of excess fluids and toxins from the body.

How to Use: Add fresh parsley to your diet (such as in salads or smoothies), or drink parsley tea to support kidney detox.

Digestive Health

Ginger:

Benefits: Ginger stimulates digestion and can help relieve bloating, indigestion, and nausea. It also promotes the detoxification of the gastrointestinal system.

How to Use: Drink ginger tea (1-2 cups daily) or add fresh ginger to meals to aid digestion and detoxify the digestive tract.

Apple Cider Vinegar:

Benefits: Apple cider vinegar (ACV) supports digestion, balances pH levels, and promotes the elimination of toxins from the body. It may also help reduce bloating and improve gut health.

How to Use: Dilute 1-2 tablespoons of apple cider vinegar in a glass of water and drink it before meals to aid digestion and detoxification.

Antioxidants and Phytonutrients

Green Tea:

Benefits: Green tea is rich in antioxidants like catechins, which help neutralize free radicals and support the body's detoxification processes.

How to Use: Drink 2-3 cups of green tea daily to boost antioxidant intake and support detoxification.

Turmeric:

Benefits: Turmeric contains curcumin, a potent antioxidant that helps reduce inflammation, protect liver function, and promote the removal of toxins.

How to Use: Add turmeric to meals or take turmeric supplements (typically 500-1,000 mg daily) to enhance detoxification.

Beets:

Benefits: Beets support liver detoxification and promote the elimination of toxins through the digestive system. They are also high in antioxidants and fiber.

How to Use: Drink beet juice, add beets to salads, or include roasted beets in meals to support liver and digestive health.

Skin Detoxification

Clay Masks:

Benefits: Clay masks, particularly those made from bentonite or clay rich in minerals, help draw out toxins from the skin, unclog pores, and reduce inflammation.

How to Use: Apply a clay mask to your face once or twice a week to cleanse the skin and remove impurities.

Activated Charcoal:

Benefits: Activated charcoal is known for its ability to bind to toxins and impurities, helping to cleanse the skin and digestive system.

How to Use: Use activated charcoal in skin care products or take activated charcoal supplements (typically 500-1,000 mg) for detoxification.

Sweating and Detoxification

Sauna or Steam Room:

Benefits: Sweating helps the body expel toxins through the skin, and using a sauna or steam room can enhance this process by increasing circulation and promoting sweating.

How to Use: Spend 15-20 minutes in a sauna or steam room a few times a week to promote detoxification and cleanse the body through sweating.

Exercise:

Benefits: Physical activity stimulates sweating, boosts circulation, and supports lymphatic drainage, all of which help the body eliminate toxins.

How to Use: Engage in regular exercise (such as walking, running, yoga, or strength training) to promote detoxification and overall health.

Fasting and Intermittent Fasting

Benefits: Fasting or intermittent fasting gives the digestive system time to rest, which supports the natural detoxification process. During fasting, the body can focus on repairing cells, removing toxins, and improving metabolic function.

How to Use: Consider adopting a fasting regimen such as the 16:8 method (16 hours of fasting, 8-hour eating window) or a full 24-hour fast a few times per week to promote detoxification.

Natural detoxification and cleansing strategies help support the body's innate ability to eliminate toxins, improve organ function, and restore overall vitality. While these remedies can be highly beneficial, they should complement a healthy lifestyle, which includes a nutritious diet, adequate hydration, regular exercise, and proper sleep. If you are considering a detox program or cleansing regimen, it's essential to consult with a healthcare provider to ensure it is suitable for your individual health needs.

CHAPTER 15

General Wellness and Longevity

Wellness and longevity are deeply interconnected with maintaining good physical, mental, and emotional health throughout life. While genetics play a role in lifespan, lifestyle choices have a much more significant influence on overall health and longevity. Embracing natural remedies and holistic approaches can help you maintain vitality, prevent chronic diseases, and support healthy aging.

Here are several natural strategies to promote general wellness and longevity:

Balanced Diet for Longevity
Whole Foods:
Benefits: A diet rich in whole, unprocessed foods is crucial for long-term health. These foods provide essential nutrients, fiber, and antioxidants that help fight inflammation, support the immune system, and prevent disease.
How to Use: Incorporate a variety of vegetables, fruits, whole grains, lean proteins, and healthy fats into your daily meals.

Antioxidant-Rich Foods:
Benefits: Antioxidants help combat oxidative stress, which contributes to aging and the development of chronic diseases.
How to Use: Consume foods like berries, nuts, seeds, leafy greens, dark chocolate, and green tea to boost antioxidant intake and support cellular health.

Omega-3 Fatty Acids:
Benefits: Omega-3 fatty acids are essential for heart health, reducing inflammation, and improving brain function.

How to Use: Include fatty fish like salmon, mackerel, and sardines in your diet, or take omega-3 supplements (typically 1,000-3,000 mg daily) if you don't consume enough fish.

Fiber-Rich Foods:
Benefits: Fiber supports digestive health, lowers cholesterol levels, and helps regulate blood sugar.
How to Use: Add fiber-rich foods like beans, lentils, oats, fruits, and vegetables to your diet to promote digestive health and longevity.

Regular Physical Activity
Aerobic Exercise:
Benefits: Regular aerobic exercise improves cardiovascular health, increases lifespan, and supports weight management. It helps keep the heart, lungs, and blood vessels in optimal condition.
How to Use: Aim for at least 150 minutes of moderate-intensity aerobic activity (such as walking, swimming, or cycling) each week.

Strength Training:
Benefits: Strength training helps maintain muscle mass, bone density, and joint function, which are crucial for healthy aging and independence.
How to Use: Incorporate strength training exercises (such as weightlifting or resistance bands) 2-3 times a week to improve muscle strength and support longevity.

Flexibility and Balance:
Benefits: Flexibility exercises and balance training help prevent falls, enhance mobility, and maintain independence as you age.
How to Use: Practice yoga, Pilates, or Tai Chi to improve flexibility, coordination, and overall vitality.

Mental and Emotional Well-Being
Stress Management:
Benefits: Chronic stress is linked to a variety of health problems, including heart disease, digestive issues, and mental health disorders. Managing stress is key to maintaining wellness and longevity.
How to Use: Practice stress-reducing techniques like mindfulness meditation, deep breathing exercises, or spending time in nature to lower cortisol levels and improve mental clarity.

Social Connections:
Benefits: Strong social relationships and connections with others have been linked to increased life expectancy, better mental health, and a greater sense of purpose.
How to Use: Foster relationships with friends, family, and your community. Join social clubs, volunteer, or engage in activities that encourage connection with others.

Positive Thinking and Gratitude:
Benefits: Practicing gratitude and maintaining a positive outlook on life has been shown to improve emotional well-being and reduce the risk of chronic diseases.
How to Use: Practice daily gratitude by writing down things you're thankful for, or focus on positive aspects of life to enhance overall well-being and longevity.

Mindfulness and Meditation:
Benefits: Mindfulness practices help to reduce stress, improve focus, and promote relaxation. Meditation can also improve cognitive function and lower the risk of age-related diseases.
How to Use: Set aside time for daily meditation or mindfulness practices (10-20 minutes) to calm the mind and reduce stress.

Sleep and Rest
Quality Sleep:
Benefits: Quality sleep is essential for the body to repair itself, consolidate memories, and maintain optimal health. Poor sleep is linked to a range of health issues, including cardiovascular disease, obesity, and cognitive decline.
How to Use: Aim for 7-9 hours of uninterrupted sleep each night. Create a sleep-friendly environment by limiting screen time before bed, maintaining a consistent sleep schedule, and keeping your room cool and dark.

Sleep Hygiene Practices:
Benefits: Proper sleep hygiene helps improve sleep quality and duration, leading to better mental and physical health.
How to Use: Practice good sleep hygiene by avoiding caffeine and heavy meals before bedtime, establishing a relaxing bedtime routine, and reducing stress before sleep.

Detoxification and Cleansing
Liver Support:
Benefits: The liver plays a vital role in detoxifying the body, so supporting liver health can aid in longevity.
How to Use: Incorporate liver-supporting herbs like milk thistle, dandelion root, and turmeric, as well as antioxidant-rich foods to promote liver health and detoxification.

Colon Health:
Benefits: A healthy digestive system helps eliminate toxins from the body, supporting overall wellness.
How to Use: Eat fiber-rich foods (like fruits, vegetables, and whole grains), stay hydrated, and include probiotics (such as fermented foods) in your diet to support gut health and longevity.

Hydration:

Benefits: Proper hydration helps the body eliminate toxins through the kidneys and promotes overall health.
How to Use: Drink plenty of water throughout the day, aiming for at least 8 glasses (2 liters) daily. Adding lemon or cucumber to your water can further enhance detoxification.

Hormonal Balance
Adaptogens:
Benefits: Adaptogenic herbs like ashwagandha, rhodiola, and ginseng help balance hormones, reduce stress, and support overall vitality.
How to Use: Take adaptogenic herbs as supplements or in tea form to help regulate stress hormones and enhance energy levels.

Healthy Fats:
Benefits: Healthy fats from sources like avocados, olive oil, and nuts support hormone production and overall cell function.
How to Use: Include healthy fats in your diet to support hormone balance and maintain energy levels.

Skin and Aging
Anti-Aging Skincare:
Benefits: Skin health is an important aspect of overall wellness, and maintaining healthy, youthful skin contributes to a sense of well-being.
How to Use: Use natural oils like argan oil, rosehip oil, and coconut oil to moisturize and protect the skin. Regularly apply sunscreen to prevent sun damage and premature aging.

Collagen Support:
Benefits: Collagen is essential for skin elasticity and joint health, and its production decreases with age.

How to Use: Take collagen supplements or consume collagen-rich foods like bone broth, chicken skin, and fish to support skin and joint health.

Purpose and Fulfillment
Finding Purpose:
Benefits: Having a sense of purpose in life is strongly associated with longevity and improved mental health. People with a clear sense of purpose tend to live longer, happier lives.
How to Use: Engage in activities that provide fulfillment, such as pursuing a passion, volunteering, learning new skills, or helping others. A sense of contribution and connection boosts overall well-being.

Lifelong Learning:
Benefits: Continuous learning stimulates the brain, promotes cognitive function, and prevents mental decline.
How to Use: Stay mentally active by reading, learning new skills, or engaging in intellectually stimulating activities to support brain health and longevity.

Promoting general wellness and longevity is not just about adopting specific remedies but creating a balanced lifestyle that nurtures the body, mind, and spirit. By focusing on a healthy diet, regular exercise, mental well-being, adequate sleep, and stress management, you can enhance your quality of life and increase your chances of living a long, healthy, and fulfilling life. These natural approaches are designed to work in harmony with your body's natural processes, supporting your long-term vitality and wellness.

CHAPTER 16
Conclusion

Natural remedies offer a holistic approach to enhancing overall health, preventing illness, and promoting longevity. By incorporating nature's healing tools—such as herbs, healthy foods, exercise, and mindfulness—into your daily routine, you support your body's ability to thrive and heal naturally. These remedies not only help maintain physical health but also promote mental and emotional well-being, leading to a balanced and fulfilling life.

Integrating Natural Remedies into Daily Life

Integrating natural remedies into your daily life is a gradual process that involves adopting small, sustainable changes. Here are a few tips for incorporating them effectively:

Start Small: Begin with simple remedies like drinking herbal teas, eating more whole foods, or practicing short mindfulness exercises daily.

Create a Routine: Establish a wellness routine that includes regular physical activity, hydration, and healthy eating. This helps your body function at its best.

Consistency is Key: The benefits of natural remedies build over time. Consistency in habits like taking herbs or maintaining a regular sleep schedule will yield the best results for long-term wellness.

Listen to Your Body: Pay attention to how your body responds to different remedies. Adjust your approach based on how you feel and what works best for you.

When to Seek Professional Help

While natural remedies can be incredibly effective, there are situations where professional medical advice or intervention is necessary. Here are a few instances when it's important to consult with a healthcare provider:

Chronic or Severe Health Conditions: If you have a serious or ongoing medical condition, such as diabetes, heart disease, or a severe autoimmune disorder, always seek professional guidance before making changes to your treatment regimen.
Unexpected Side Effects: If you experience any adverse reactions to natural remedies, such as allergies or digestive discomfort, it's important to consult with a doctor or qualified health practitioner.
Emergencies: In cases of acute or life-threatening health issues (e.g., severe pain, injury, or sudden illness), always seek immediate medical attention.
Natural remedies should complement, not replace, professional care when needed. It's always wise to have open communication with your healthcare provider when incorporating new treatments into your routine, especially if you are on prescription medications or have existing health concerns.

Building a Natural First Aid Kit
A well-stocked natural first aid kit can help you address common ailments and injuries using natural remedies. Here's how to build one:

Herbal Remedies:
Chamomile Tea: For calming anxiety, promoting relaxation, or easing digestive discomfort.
Lavender Oil: For soothing skin irritations, minor burns, or promoting restful sleep.
Ginger: For nausea, digestive upset, and reducing inflammation.

Essential Oils:

Peppermint Oil: For headaches, muscle pain, and digestive issues (such as nausea or bloating).
Tea Tree Oil: For treating minor cuts, scrapes, and skin infections due to its antibacterial properties.
Eucalyptus Oil: For respiratory issues, such as colds or coughs, or muscle aches.

Supplements and Nutrients:
Vitamin C: For immune support, especially during flu season.
Probiotics: For digestive health and maintaining a healthy gut flora.
Magnesium: For muscle cramps, relaxation, and supporting sleep.

Topical Remedies:
Aloe Vera Gel: For sunburns, burns, and skin irritations.
Arnica Cream: For bruises, sprains, and muscle soreness.
Honey: For wound healing, as it has natural antimicrobial properties.

First Aid Basics:
Bandages and Gauze: For minor cuts and scrapes.
Ice Pack or Cold Compress: For swelling or inflammation.
Activated Charcoal: For detoxing or in cases of mild poisoning (consult with a healthcare provider).

Herbal Teas:
Peppermint Tea: For indigestion or nausea.
Ginger Tea: For digestive issues or to soothe inflammation.
Lemon Balm Tea: For calming anxiety or insomnia.
By keeping these natural remedies on hand, you can address common health issues and minor injuries using safe, effective, and natural methods. However, always ensure that you have access to professional medical care for more serious conditions or if natural remedies are not sufficient.

In summary, natural remedies can be powerful tools for enhancing wellness, preventing illness, and supporting longevity. By thoughtfully integrating them into daily life, being mindful of when professional help is necessary, and maintaining a natural first aid kit, you can take charge of your health and live a long, vibrant life.